American College of Physicians

of Physicians

PARKINSON'S DISEASE

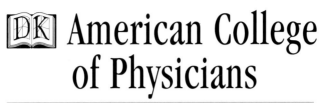

American College of Physicians

PARKINSON'S DISEASE

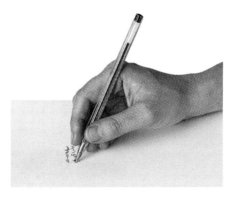

MEDICAL EDITOR
DAVID R. GOLDMANN, MD
ASSOCIATE MEDICAL EDITOR
DAVID A. HOROWITZ, MD

A DORLING KINDERSLEY BOOK

IMPORTANT

The American College of
Physicians (ACP) Home Medical
Guides provide general
information on a wide range of
health and medical topics. These
books are not substitutes for
medical diagnosis, and you should
always consult your doctor on
personal health matters before
undertaking any program of
therapy or treatment. Various
medical organizations have
different guidelines for diagnosis
and treatment of the same
conditions; the American College
of Physicians–American Society of
Internal Medicine (ACP–ASIM)
has tried to present a reasonable
consensus of these opinions.

Material in this book was
reviewed by the ACP–ASIM for
general medical accuracy and
applicability in the United States;
however, the information provided
herein does not necessarily reflect
the specific recommendations
or opinions of the ACP–ASIM.
The naming of any organization,
product, or alternative therapy in
these books is not an ACP–ASIM
endorsement, and the omission of
any such name does not indicate
ACP–ASIM disapproval.

DORLING KINDERSLEY

LONDON, NEW YORK, AUCKLAND, DELHI,
JOHANNESBURG, MUNICH, PARIS, AND SYDNEY

DK www.dk.com

Senior Editors Jill Hamilton, Nicki Lampon
Senior Designer Jan English
DTP Design Jason Little
Editor Ashley Ren
Medical Consultant Matthew Stern, MD

Senior Managing Editor Martyn Page
Senior Managing Art Editor Bryn Walls

Published in the United States in 2000 by
Dorling Kindersley Publishing, Inc.
95 Madison Avenue, New York, New York 10016

2 4 6 8 10 9 7 5 3 1

Library of Congress Catalog Card Number 99-76856
ISBN 0-7894-4169-1

Reproduced by Colourscan, Singapore
Printed and bound in the United States by Quebecor World, Taunton, Massachusetts

Contents

INTRODUCTION   7

CAUSES AND CHARACTERISTICS   11

TYPES OF PARKINSONISM   18

SYMPTOMS AND SIGNS   22

HOW IS THE DIAGNOSIS MADE?   28

DOES PARKINSON'S DISEASE AFFECT THE MIND?   32

DISABILITY IN PARKINSON'S DISEASE   39

MEDICAL TREATMENT   44

SURGERY FOR PARKINSON'S DISEASE   59

GENERAL MANAGEMENT   62

QUESTIONS AND ANSWERS   71

USEFUL ADDRESSES   73

NOTES   74

INDEX   78

ACKNOWLEDGMENTS   80

Introduction

If you, or a close relative or friend, suffer from Parkinson's disease, this book is written for you. It is designed to help you understand the symptoms and disabilities caused by the disease and to suggest what you can do for yourself as well as what doctors can do to treat the condition.

The good news is that, although there is still much to be learned about Parkinson's disease, the grim prospects that prevailed 30 years ago have been much improved by increased understanding and modern forms of treatment.

AN IMPROVED OUTLOOK
Modern treatments mean that people with Parkinson's disease can now enjoy a much more active life than did sufferers in previous decades.

▬ WHAT IS PARKINSON'S DISEASE? ▬

Parkinson's disease is characterized by a collection of symptoms involving the nervous system, the most important of which are:

- Slowness of movement.
- Rigidity, which makes the limbs feel heavy and stiff.
- Shaking of the hands and sometimes the legs at rest.
- Posture disorders, in which the patient's neck and trunk assume a bent position and the arms fail to swing freely when the patient is walking.

Parkinson's disease is caused by the degeneration of pigmented nerve cells in the brain. The disease usually starts in the 50s or 60s and may not worsen for months or even years, but it usually progresses. However, Parkinson's disease seldom shortens life expectancy to any significant degree.

In the advanced stages, tremor, slowness, and rigidity may affect all four limbs and the trunk. Speech may be indistinct and slurred, the limbs and body are bent, and the patient is apt to walk with short, stumbling steps and is prone to falling.

WHO GETS IT?

Parkinson's disease may afflict people from all classes of society, from all ethnic groups, and occurs throughout the world.

It progresses with age, but is not caused by aging itself. Overall, approximately one person in 1,000 is affected, but the proportion increases to about one in 100 for people in their 70s and 80s.

Many elderly people are so mildly affected by Parkinson's disease that it is easily overlooked.

Men and women are equally affected by Parkinson's disease, and the disease is seldom inherited.

DON'T GET TOO DEPRESSED

If this description sounds depressing, remember that for many years the disability is mild, and during this time most patients are capable of normal domestic activities and can usually continue their regular employment.

Furthermore, although there is no cure for Parkinson's disease at the present time, many of the symptoms can be well controlled by appropriate treatment.

How Is the Diagnosis Made?

People wonder how the diagnosis is made. It is invariably a clinical decision, based on the symptoms and especially the signs that an experienced doctor can observe during an examination.

Laboratory tests and X-rays are unnecessary for diagnosis of Parkinson's disease in most cases, and special tests such as computerized tomography (CT) scanning and magnetic resonance imaging (MRI) are usually not helpful. Indeed, such scans often do not reveal an abnormality in people with Parkinson's disease.

How Is It Treated?

Treatment is based on the replacement of those chemicals in the brain that are reduced or depleted by Parkinson's disease. The main chemical that is affected by the disease is dopamine, which diminishes slowly over a number of years before any symptoms become apparent.

It is estimated that you have to lose a significant proportion of the dopamine in the critical areas of your brain before symptoms or signs are evident. Dopamine is found in groups of nerve cells in the base of the brain, called the basal ganglia.

Patients are given a drug called levodopa to replace the missing dopamine, but other drugs are used as well, often to enhance the effect of levodopa.

Physical, speech, and occupational therapy can all be valuable at certain stages of Parkinson's disease. These supplement drug treatment but are not an effective substitute for it. The aim throughout treatment is to maintain your mobility and allow you to pursue as normal a lifestyle as possible.

WHO WILL TREAT YOU?

Patients and their families have to be as involved as the doctors and therapists. Your primary care physician may be the first person you consult and indeed may assume responsibility for managing your condition, including making the diagnosis, explaining and prescribing drugs, and possibly organizing physical and occupational therapy. Ideally, a neurologist, preferably one with special training or an interest in Parkinson's disease, will assume your care. Often, the neurologist will work with your primary care physician to provide continuing care.

KEY POINTS

- Parkinson's disease can affect people from all ethnic groups and social classes, and men and women are equally affected.
- The illness is most common in elderly people.
- Symptoms can be controlled by appropriate treatment.

Causes and characteristics

The essential cause is not known. Clues are available from studies of the distribution of the disease – that is, who is affected, where, and in what circumstances. It is relatively common, and perhaps as many as 1,000,000 patients are affected in the US at any one time. Men and women are equally affected, and no ethnic group is immune.

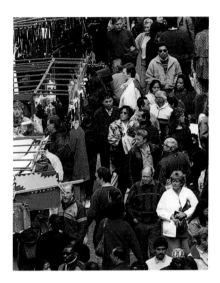

Parkinson's disease is not associated with any particular job and is clearly a physical disease of the brain that is not caused by stress, anxiety, or family problems. Extensive searches for a viral or bacterial cause for the condition have thus far proved negative.

DEMOCRATIC DISEASE
Parkinson's disease is equally common among men and women and does not affect one occupation or ethnic group more than another.

NERVE CELL DEGENERATION

In patients who have Parkinson's disease, there is disease or degeneration of the so-called basal ganglia in the deeper gray matter of the brain, particularly of that part known as the substantia nigra.

The Function of the Substantia Nigra

Nerve cells in the substantia nigra, in the upper part of the brain stem, contain the neurotransmitter dopamine. Nerve fibers in these cells release dopamine into the corpus striatum, a part of the brain that controls movement.

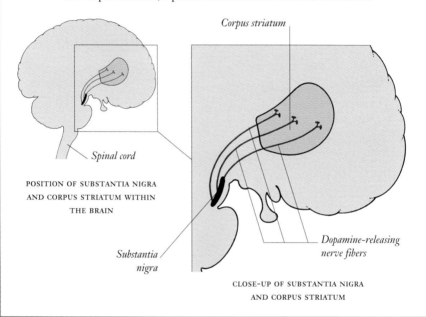

Corpus striatum

Spinal cord

POSITION OF SUBSTANTIA NIGRA
AND CORPUS STRIATUM WITHIN
THE BRAIN

Substantia nigra

Dopamine-releasing nerve fibers

CLOSE-UP OF SUBSTANTIA NIGRA
AND CORPUS STRIATUM

The substantia nigra, which is connected to the corpus striatum (caudate nucleus and globus pallidus), contains black pigmented cells and, in normal individuals, produces a number of chemical transmitters, the most important of which is dopamine. Other transmitters include serotonin, somatostatin, and norepinephrine. In Parkinson's disease, the basal ganglia cells produce less dopamine, which is needed to transmit vital messages to other parts of the brain and to the spinal cord, nerves, and muscles.

The basal ganglia, through the action of dopamine, are responsible for planning and controlling automatic movements of the body, such as pointing, pulling on a sock, writing, and walking. If the basal ganglia are not working properly, as in patients with Parkinson's disease, all aspects of movement are impaired, resulting in the characteristic features of the disease: slowness of movement, stiffness and effort required to move a limb, and often tremor.

Dopamine levels in the brain's substantia nigra do decrease naturally with aging. However, they have to fall significantly below normal values for the symptoms and signs of parkinsonism to emerge.

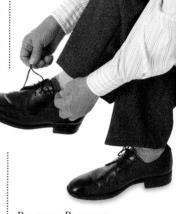

PRACTICAL PROBLEMS
People with Parkinson's disease find their movements become slow and stiff, and they have problems with routine tasks such as tying shoelaces.

RESTORING THE BALANCE

Normally, there is an even balance between dopamine and another neurotransmitter known as acetylcholine.

How Drug Treatment Works

Brain-cell degeneration in Parkinson's disease cannot be stopped, but drugs can minimize the effects for years. They help restore the balance between dopamine and acetylcholine by boosting dopamine levels and inactivating some acetylcholine.

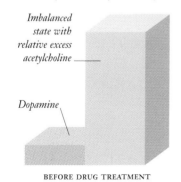

Imbalanced state with relative excess acetylcholine

Dopamine

BEFORE DRUG TREATMENT

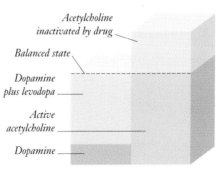

Acetylcholine inactivated by drug

Balanced state

Dopamine plus levodopa

Active acetylcholine

Dopamine

AFTER DRUG TREATMENT

Acetylcholine is present in many areas of the brain and plays a part in normal memory recording and recall. Since dopamine is depleted, there is a relative excess of acetylcholine. Therefore, two groups of drugs used to treat Parkinson's disease are dopamine drugs (levodopa) and anticholinergics, which are drugs designed to restore the balance by diminishing the acetylcholine. Recent studies have implicated other neurotransmitters in Parkinson's disease, and newer therapies act on these other systems, such as GABA and serotonin.

How Do Nerve Cells Send Messages?

The diagram (opposite) shows how a nerve cell, or neuron, in the basal ganglia transmits an impulse down its main wire, or axon, to the synaptic knob, which releases a package of dopamine. When this passes into receptors of the next nerve cell, it transmits the message further down the line. This process is carried out by millions of neurons at the same time, forming a network of activity far exceeding that of the telephone company.

Current ideas about the cause of Parkinson's disease suggest that some people are born with a predisposition that makes them vulnerable to some unidentified environmental toxic agents. Why cells die in the substantia nigra of patients with Parkinson's disease is unknown. This important group of cells shows three changes:

• Evidence of oxidative stress, in which the release of oxygen by cells damages the cells and depletes their level of the protein glutathione.

• High levels of iron.

• A deficiency of an essential component of all body cells (mitochondrial complex 1) that normally controls oxidative reactions.

How Dopamine Conducts Nerve Impulses

When electrical impulses passing along the axon of a nerve cell reach the synaptic knob, stored dopamine is released. This passes across the gap, or synapse, to receptors in the next nerve cell, causing an impulse to pass along the second cell.

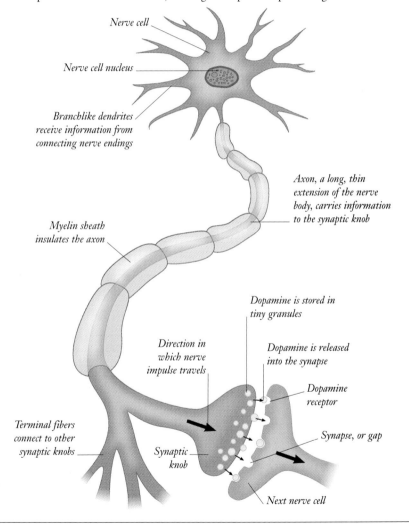

Nerve cell

Nerve cell nucleus

Branchlike dendrites receive information from connecting nerve endings

Axon, a long, thin extension of the nerve body, carries information to the synaptic knob

Myelin sheath insulates the axon

Dopamine is stored in tiny granules

Direction in which nerve impulse travels

Dopamine is released into the synapse

Dopamine receptor

Terminal fibers connect to other synaptic knobs

Synaptic knob

Synapse, or gap

Next nerve cell

15

It is not known which of the three changes is the primary event that causes the secondary changes culminating in substantia nigral cell death. In people who have not yet developed symptoms but have the early brain changes of Parkinson's disease, the substantia nigra shows a comparable loss of reduced glutathione and possibly a reduction of complex 1 activity as well. These abnormalities provide a new focus for the development of future treatments.

The dopamine receptors are most important. Some drugs, such as major tranquilizers, can block the receptors and, if taken for a long period, they block the passage of dopamine in the nerve cells and their connecting network of axons. The nerve impulses, so essential for normal movement, are therefore reduced. This is the basis of the drug-induced parkinsonism described in the next chapter.

AGING AND HEREDITY

Although Parkinson's disease is *not* caused by the normal aging process that affects our brains and other organs, incidence of the disease does increase with age. A family history of the disease occurs in 5–10 percent of patients, but studies that have been done on twins suggest that hereditary factors are, in fact, relatively unimportant. Affected relatives may share exposure to some as yet unknown environmental agent or they may be genetically vulnerable to it.

KEY POINTS

- The cause of Parkinson's disease is unknown.
- Research has shown that pigment-containing cells in the deep part of the brain that produce dopamine and other important chemicals degenerate and die. The loss of these cells, in turn, affects the working of other parts of the brain and the spinal cord, nerves, and muscles involved in movement.
- When the chemical dopamine is depleted, there is a relative excess of the chemical acetylcholine.
- Treatment is aimed at boosting dopamine levels and/or diminishing acetylcholine levels.

Types of parkinsonism

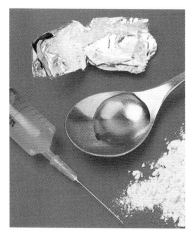

We distinguish Parkinson's disease (idiopathic Parkinson's disease or paralysis agitans), described by James Parkinson in 1817, from a group of rarer disorders also caused by impairment of the function of the nerve cells of the brain and called secondary or symptomatic parkinsonism.

AN EFFECT OF DRUG ABUSE
A chemical that is found in drugs used by heroin addicts has been found to cause symptomatic parkinsonism very quickly.

There are several kinds of symptomatic parkinsonism:
- Drug-induced parkinsonism.
- Postencephalitic parkinsonism.
- Poison-induced parkinsonism.
- Multiple-system atrophies.

It is important that the doctor distinguishes between true Parkinson's disease and symptomatic parkinsonism, because the treatment may be quite different.

DRUG-INDUCED

Neuroleptic drugs used in the treatment of schizophrenia and other serious psychotic mental illnesses can block dopamine receptors in the substantia nigra and corpus striatum, and thereby produce symptoms that mimic Parkinson's disease. The most common neuroleptic drugs are the phenothiazines, but there are many others, as shown in the table on page 20. The list is not complete and, if in doubt, you should ask your primary care physician or your specialist if the drug you are taking might cause parkinsonism.

Some of these drugs are used to counter nausea, vomiting, or dizziness and, under these circumstances, parkinsonism should not develop if the course of treatment is restricted to less than a month. If it is possible for for your physician to withdraw the drugs, the parkinsonism will usually slowly disappear, although this may take several months. Some patients with serious psychiatric illness need to continue the neuroleptic drugs; some degree of parkinsonism then has to be tolerated to maintain mental stability and can usually be controlled.

POSTENCEPHALITIC

This type of parkinsonism is now extremely rare. It developed in the wake of a diffuse inflammation of the brain (encephalitis) caused by an epidemic of a particular viral infection that raged throughout the world between 1918 and 1926. The symptoms and treatment are slightly different from those of idiopathic Parkinson's disease.

POISON-INDUCED

It has been found that meperidine hydrochloride (MPTP), a chemical contaminant of recreational drugs made illegally and used by heroin addicts, mainly in California, can produce parkinsonism within days or weeks. Brains examined after death in such cases show severe destruction of the substantia nigra and profound loss of dopamine and other neural transmitters, as is seen in Parkinson's disease.

Drugs that Can Cause Parkinsonism

Below is a list of neuroleptic drugs used in the treatment of serious psychiatric illnesses such as schizophrenia that have been known to cause symptomatic parkinsonism.

COMMONLY USED NEUROLEPTIC DRUGS	SIMILAR NEUROLEPTIC ANTIPSYCHOTIC DRUGS	NEUROLEPTIC DRUGS GIVEN BY INJECTION
Chlorpromazine (Thorazine)	Droperidol (Fentanyl)	Fluphenazine (Fluphenazine HCl, Prolixin)
Fluphenazine (Fluphenazine HCl, Prolixin)	Haloperidol (Haldol)	Haloperidol (Haldol)
Trifluoperazine (Stelazine)	Reserpine (Diupres, Hydropres, Diutensin-R)	
Prochlorperazine (Compazine)	Pimozide (Orap)	
Thioridazine (Thioridazine HCl)	Risperidone (Risperdal)	
Perphenazine (Etrafon, Triavil, Trilafon)		

The symptoms are controlled by levodopa drugs, which replace the missing dopamine in the same way as in Parkinson's disease. However, the brain damage inflicted by MPTP is permanent. Researchers now know that certain poisons can damage the brain in a way similar to that arising spontaneously in idiopathic

Parkinson's disease, a valuable finding for further research into the sequence of events leading to degeneration of the dopamine-generating cells. For example, in animals in which parkinsonism is artificially induced by injecting MPTP, the dopamine-producing cells in the substantia nigra are deficient in one of the important enzymes, complex 1, which is involved in oxygen control in the cell. These studies are providing important clues to human disease and strategies for novel therapies. However, in spite of improved knowledge and understanding of the nature and causes of Parkinson's disease, more work needs to be done to further our knowledge and to develop better treatments.

OTHER TYPES

Parkinsonism is not usually a feature of head injury and is seldom a symptom of a brain tumor. Other disorders characterized by rigid akinetic states can be due to various degenerations of the brain, such as progressive supranuclear palsy, multiple-system atrophies, and diffuse cortical Lewy body disease. These disorders are less common causes of parkinsonism and need specialized neurological care. They do not respond well to antiparkinsonism drugs.

KEY POINT

- Various types of symptomatic parkinsonism need to be distinguished from Parkinson's disease because the treatment may be different.

Symptoms and signs

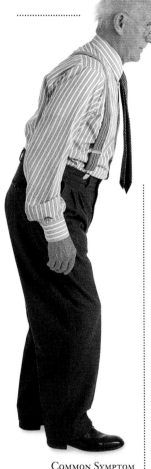

The principal physical symptoms that affect people suffering from Parkinson's disease are tremor, muscular rigidity, akinesia, abnormal posture, and loss of balance.

Let's examine the symptoms and signs of Parkinson's disease in greater detail, although we must always bear in mind that different patients will experience these to varying degrees. In addition, the physical manifestations of Parkinson's disease, both symptoms and signs, usually change in the individual over time. For example, your movements may be visibly slow (bradykinesia). You may rise slowly from a chair or walk slowly with short steps. You may have a slow rhythmic tremor of one or both hands that disappears when you grasp a chair or take hold of an object. Many years ago, this tremor was compared to rolling pills made by hand and was therefore called a "pill-rolling tremor." When the doctor bends or straightens your wrist or arm or leg, he or she may feel a resistance as if trying to bend a lead pipe. The tremor may also seem superimposed on the rigidity, creating a sensation of turning a cogwheel, known as cogwheel rigidity.

COMMON SYMPTOM
Patients often tend to lean forward from their center of gravity when they walk.

22

TREMOR

The most common early symptom is shaking (tremor) of one or both hands. Tremor occurs at rest and is reduced or stopped when the imb is in action. It usually vanishes during sleep. Tremor is fairly slow, about five beats per second, and is rhythmical.

RIGIDITY

As a result of rigidity, felt as stiffness, a sense of effort is required for a patient with Parkinson's disease to move his or her limbs because they may feel heavy and weak. However, loss of muscle strength and power is not a feature of Parkinson's disease.

SLOW MOVEMENT

Slowness of movement can be experienced in three ways: lack of spontaneous movement (akinesia), slowness in starting to move, and slowness during the movement itself (bradykinesia, *brady*: slow, *kinesis*: movement). Handwriting tends to become progressively smaller (known as micrographia, from the Latin *micro*: small, and *graphos*: writing), and the writing may show signs of the tremor.

DISORDER OF POSTURE

Disorder of posture is the term that refers to the bent position of the neck and trunk that develops late in the

Common Symptoms of Parkinson's Disease

Although the symptoms of Parkinson's disease vary from patient to patient, there is a range of common characteristics.

- Difficulty fastening buttons
- Inability to turn over
- Inability to get up from a chair
- Expressionless face
- Frequent falls
- Feet become immobile
- Oily skin
- Blinking only rarely
- Shuffling steps
- Slow eating
- Slow movement
- Soft voice
- Stiff limbs
- Tremor

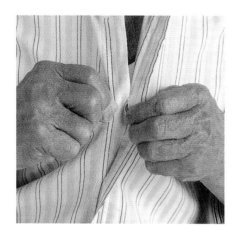

DRESSING DIFFICULTIES
Stiffness and slow movement can cause difficulty in fastening buttons, making dressing frustrating.

disease. It describes the way the arms are held close to the sides, elbows and wrists slightly bent. The legs, too, may be flexed at the hips and knees.

LOSS OF BALANCE
Loss of balance often accompanies disordered posture but is usually a later feature. Patients find it difficult to correct a stumble (lack of righting reflexes) and are likely to fall. They lean forward in front of their center of gravity and, without being able to help themselves, a walk may break into a run (called festination, from the Latin *festinare*, to hasten). Or, if pushed gently, patients may run forward or stumble backward uncontrollably.

CHANGED BLADDER AND BOWEL HABITS
Constipation is an almost inevitable symptom of Parkinson's disease. It may be caused by sluggish movement of the muscles in the bowel or by the antiparkinson medications themselves. Although constipation is not a serious symptom, it does cause concern and apprehension, especially in the elderly.

The bladder muscle also contracts less efficiently and, as a result, frequent urination is common, with small volumes and some degree of urgency. In older men, coincidental enlargement of the prostate may add to the problems, causing a slow urine stream in addition to a need to get up at night to urinate.

If you suffer from constipation or frequent urination, you may need to be assessed by both a neurologist and a urologist. Incontinence does not occur in the early stages of Parkinson's disease, and if it does occur later, it may have some other cause. You may have accidents as a result of moving too slowly to get to the toilet on time. This is known as urge incontinence, rather than true incontinence, and it can sometimes be improved by treatment with medications such as oxybutynin.

SWALLOWING DIFFICULTIES

Occasionally, difficulty swallowing develops as a result of Parkinson's disease, but special tests are required to make sure that this symptom is not due to some other cause that may have arisen by chance.

AUTOMATIC MOVEMENTS

Actions are noticeably labored. Most of us perform automatic movements unconsciously at rest when sitting comfortably. Movements such as blinking, crossing and uncrossing the legs, and fidgeting, for example, are lacking in the Parkinson's disease patient. When walking, Parkinson's disease patients often use short steps and shuffle as if their feet are glued to the floor. Their gait is hesitant, and their steps shorten even more in doorways, when there is an obstruction, or if a dog or a stranger runs across their path. Sometimes patients get stuck when walking; their feet feel frozen to the ground. If this sensation happens to you, it is often effective to focus on a spot in front of you and aim at it with the leading leg. You will generally find that you can start to walk again.

FACIAL APPEARANCE AND SPEECH

The face may lack expression, the eyes are a little fixed, and in advanced cases of Parkinson's disease, there is a tendency to drool. This arises not because of excessive saliva formation, but because of reduction in the normal swallowing of saliva that we do unconsciously and automatically. The voice is quiet, sometimes hoarse (dysphonia), and speech may be slurred (dysarthria). These problems may be inconspicuous but may manifest themselves as difficulty singing.

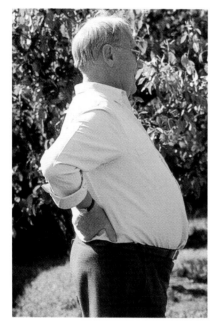

STIFFNESS IN THE BACK
Sufferers sometimes experience aching and stiffness in the back, neck, and limbs, making movement difficult.

OTHER PROBLEMS

Usually, other problems are late features that appear many years after Parkinson's disease is first diagnosed. Most patients are able to walk well, speak clearly, and work and enjoy leisure activities for many years. Modern treatments can control symptoms effectively in most sufferers.

Other problems are also occasionally troublesome for patients. Pain is not a serious problem for most sufferers, although aching and stiffness in the neck, back, and limbs is quite common. A stiff or frozen shoulder may develop as a result of reduced automatic movement. This is painful and prevents men from getting to their wallets in their back trouser pockets, and it causes difficulties for women with their zippers and bra fasteners. These incidental problems can be treated effectively.

Occasionally, patients are affected by writer's cramp. Drug side effects can also cause symptoms.

KEY POINTS

- Symptoms of Parkinson's disease include tremor, rigidity, akinesia, posture disorders, and loss of balance.
- Symptoms vary a great deal and, later in the illness, may include difficulty swallowing and changed bladder and bowel habits.
- Signs include reduced automatic movements, altered facial appearance, and speech difficulties.

How is the diagnosis made?

Some patients and their relatives worry about the accuracy of the diagnosis. One patient differs from the next, and your symptoms and appearance may be different from those of that man you have seen shaking in your local store, who is said to have Parkinson's disease. In most cases, however, an accurate diagnosis is not difficult.

MAKING A DIAGNOSIS
Although there are no clinical tests to confirm a diagnosis, the signs and symptoms of Parkinson's disease are usually easy for an expert to detect.

As with certain other diseases, no specific or diagnostic tests exist that either confirm or exclude a diagnosis of Parkinson's disease. The results of blood tests, electro-encephalograms (EEG), computerized tomography (CT) scanning, and magnetic resonance imaging (MRI) are all essentially normal.

Parkinson's disease can be mistaken for other diseases, and, because the outlook and treatment may be substantially different, it is generally advisable for the initial suspicion to be confirmed or rejected by a neurologist.

The diagnosis is based on the history and signs and, to the expert eye, it may be immediately evident when the patient enters the examination room. A change in handwriting, dragging of one leg in the absence of hip disease, or a complaint of clumsiness will all alert the primary care physician to the possible diagnosis of Parkinson's disease. The severity and the type of illness will be explored during the clinical examination and the degree of disability will be determined through questioning about what you can and cannot do.

Diseases with Similar Signs

You can see from the tables on page 30 that there are other causes of shaking and tremors that can be mistaken for Parkinson's disease.

The most frequent cause of shaking and tremors is a common condition called benign essential tremor, which occurs in about 2–4 percent of the population in varying degrees. In this condition, the shaking is slight or absent at rest but worse when the arms are held stretched out. There is usually no rigidity or slowness of movement and also no tendency to a bent or flexed posture. Benign essential tremor often, but not always, runs in families, and the tremor may be reduced by a small dose of alcohol. This condition does not respond to antiparkinsonism drugs.

Thyroid disease, alcoholism, severe depression, and a variety of rare metabolic and structural disorders can occasionally mimic Parkinson's disease, but the doctor will consider these disorders when he or she is making the evaluation.

SHARED SYMPTOM
Diseases such as benign essential tremor can also cause handwriting to become shaky, but in Parkinson's disease the writing also becomes smaller.

Conditions with Symptoms like Those of Parkinson's Disease

A number of neurological diseases produce physical symptoms that may mimic Parkinson's disease.

- Postencephalitic parkinsonism; drug-induced parkinsonism.
- Other causes of tremor such as benign essential tremor, hyperthyroidism, or alcoholism.
- Other brain diseases such as multiple strokes.

Diseases that People Commonly Confuse with Parkinson's Disease

Parkinson's disease is sometimes confused with other, unrelated conditions, some of which can produce similar symptoms.

- Brain tumor
- Strokes
- Aftereffects of head injury
- Multiple sclerosis
- Alzheimer's disease and primary dementia
- Motor neuron disease

MULTIPLE SCLEROSIS AND STROKES

Occasionally, people who are subsequently diagnosed as having Parkinson's disease wonder if it could be multiple sclerosis or some unusual form of stroke. However, multiple sclerosis is mainly a disease of younger people, and its symptoms and signs are quite different and can be quickly recognized by a specialist.

Multiple strokes affecting in turn each side of the body can produce a picture that superficially resembles

Parkinson's disease; but here too, specialists can distinguish between the two conditions. Of course, both conditions can arise by chance in the same person, but a neurologist can usually clarify the issue. Strokes do not, however, cause Parkinson's disease.

ALZHEIMER'S DISEASE

Sometimes the more advanced or elderly patient may suffer from memory loss or develop periods of confusion. The family rightly asks, "Is he becoming demented?" "Is he developing Alzheimer's disease?" Patients with Alzheimer's disease and those with diffuse cortical Lewy body disease, which is superficially similar, have mental symptoms of forgetfulness and poor judgment from the beginning, whereas in Parkinson's disease the early symptoms are physical slowness, stiffness, or tremor. Although some of the symptoms of Alzheimer's and Parkinson's disease overlap and resemble each other, neurologists can usually distinguish these conditions on clinical evidence, supplemented as needed by brain scans and other tests.

KEY POINTS

- In most cases, an accurate diagnosis is not difficult.
- Parkinson's disease should not be confused with, and is not caused by, multiple sclerosis or strokes.
- People with Alzheimer's disease have mental symptoms from the beginning, whereas the early symptoms in Parkinson's disease are physical slowness, stiffness, or tremor.

Does Parkinson's disease affect the mind?

*N*erves and emotional factors play
their part in all human disease. The
effects of worry and sleeplessness
in worsening the pain of even
a minor bruise or a toothache
are as well known as the
harmful effects of worry on
the symptoms of asthma
or a stomach ulcer.

EMOTIONAL EFFECTS
*Feeling dependent on others
may cause anxiety and
depression in the Parkinson's
disease sufferer.*

Understandably, if you have
a physical illness such as
bronchitis, a breast lump, a
broken leg, or Parkinson's
disease, it is not surprising
that you feel somewhat anxious, apprehensive, or even
depressed about your condition.

The most obvious psychological accompaniments of
Parkinson's disease are anxiety and depression caused by
the physical symptoms of the disease and the disability
it produces. Tremor and ponderous slow movements

are a source of social embarrassment. An abnormal or awkward gait, trips and falls, and difficulty with speech and voice also embarrass the sufferer. At a very late stage of the disease, after many years, the physical handicaps can be severe and may restrict many activities; it is no wonder, then, that patients feel despondent and depressed, particularly about their dependence on others. Fears of future incapacity add to their concerns.

DEPRESSION

A depressive illness occurs at some point in about one-half of all Parkinson's disease patients. Depressive illness here means symptoms out of proportion to the underlying cause, or symptoms of such severity that the patient cannot cope with them. Depression can occur out of the blue when there is no apparent stress, source of anxiety, or physical disability to explain it. This is called endogenous depression. It is of interest that the incidence is higher in people with Parkinson's disease, even before the physical signs are apparent, compared to the incidence in normal people.

SYMPTOMS OF DEPRESSION

If you have ever been depressed, you will remember the feelings of being miserable, unhappy, and blue. You probably also remember the apathy and being devoid of vitality, interests, and enthusiasm. Being depressed is quite different from the common complaint of being bored, anxious, or just fed up. Depressed patients have to push themselves to make the effort to do everyday tasks like getting dressed, shaving, or putting on makeup, going out, mixing socially, or even chatting with family or friends. Life seems pointless, hopeless, and

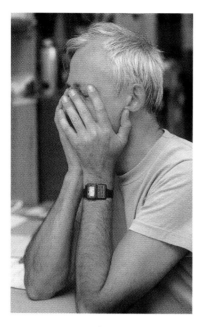

A SENSE OF HOPELESSNESS
A person with depression may feel hopeless and lifeless, and may lack the enthusiasm to do anything constructive. Depression usually responds well to treatment, however.

futile. Normal sleep patterns are disturbed. Patients go to bed early, just to get away from it all, sleep fitfully until 4 or 5 am, and then cannot sleep anymore. Early morning tends to be the worst time, and by evening the blues may have receded a little. These daily mood swings are characteristic of the disease.

Physical symptoms such as vague pains, headaches, backaches, palpitations, and often a fear of cancer may dominate their lives, adding to the mental miseries. Feelings of wholly inappropriate guilt are mixed with a sense of inadequacy. If you are depressed, you blame yourself for all your family's misfortunes and sometimes for all the evils of the world. You may feel periods of restlessness and agitation.

If you feel like this, you need medical attention. Depressed people may commit suicide, but this is fortunately rare in Parkinson's disease.

HOW IS DEPRESSION TREATED?

Symptoms of depression generally respond well to antidepressant drugs of the tricyclic group, such as amitriptyline, but they must be supervised by your primary care physician or specialist. These antidepressant drugs do not interact with antiparkinsonism drugs.

Newer antidepressant drugs are of equal value and include paroxitene (generic of Paxil), fluoxetine (generic of Prozac), or sertraline (generic of Zoloft). Treatment is usually necessary for 6–12 months and sometimes longer. In most cases, the results are good.

CONFUSION

Confusion and hallucinations are uncommon, both in younger patients and in the early stages of the disease. Do not forget that many people over the age of 70 have periods of memory lapses, disorientation, and confusion. Deafness and impaired vision can lead to hallucinations in people without Parkinson's disease. When these symptoms occur in those with Parkinson's disease, they may be the result of aging effects alone or they may be caused by drugs.

Antiparkinsonism drugs of all types may cause disorientation, confusion, and hallucinations. The most commonly used drugs are the anticholinergic drugs trihexiphenidyl, orphenadrine, and benztropine, but bromocriptine and levodopa drugs can also result in confused states.

WHAT ARE THE SIGNS OF CONFUSION?

Nightmares and frequent dreams are early warnings of these unpleasant side effects. In most instances these problems come and go intermittently, but they always tend to be more noticeable at night and in strange surroundings such as hospitals or nursing homes. Disorientation may be related to time, place, or person. The patient is bewildered and does not know where he or she is, or what time of day it is. Recent information is imperfectly registered, so that the patient may deny having had lunch an hour earlier or forget having seen a recent visitor.

Visual hallucinations consist of seeing things that are not there, such as people, faces, insects, or animals. Auditory hallucinations consist of hearing sounds or voices that are not there. Voices may seem to come from a radio or television, or they may seem to come from inside the patient's head. Sometimes the patient knows that they are unreal and has insight into these intrusions, but at other times he or she may believe them to be real. These symptoms can cause severe distress and agitation.

The patient's confusion may betray itself in peculiar conversation or strange, erratic behavior. Some individuals may wander off and get lost. They are often inattentive and easily distractable, and memory appears poor because they seem unable to concentrate. Alternatively, they might pour milk into the coffeepot, put clothes on backward, attempt to eat dessert with a knife, or find themselves unable to tie a knot or use a comb or razor. These latter difficulties are called apraxia, the inability to perform skilled movements and sequences when the limbs have normal powers of strength, coordination, and sensation.

DRUG-RELATED EFFECTS

Although these symptoms may occur in demented patients and are often not totally curable, they may just be a sign of sensitivity to drugs. The doctor will reduce or gradually taper any possible offending drug and the unpleasant symptoms that the patient has been having will usually disappear. If a patient is dependent on current doses of antiparkinsonism drugs, newer medications (for example, atypical neuroleptics such as clozapine) are available to block the hallucinogenic effects of dopaminergic medications without exacerbating the symptoms of Parkinson's disease. A fine balance of drugs, tailored to the individual's needs, will often provide a satisfactory if not perfect solution.

DEMENTIA

One of the big concerns about Parkinson's disease is that it is known to be associated with dementia, a decline in intellect, memory, and the ability to make rational decisions and judgments. This has, without doubt, been overemphasized. Many Parkinson's patients are not affected in this way and never become demented.

In later life, both Parkinson's disease and Alzheimer's disease, the most frequent cause of dementia, are common. At the age of 70, about 5–10 percent of the population shows some signs of dementia, and about half of these will suffer from Alzheimer's disease. Consequently, there is a chance that some patients have both parkinsonism and dementia purely by coincidence.

The combination of both Parkinson's disease and Alzheimer's disease is obviously unfortunate, and the outlook is considerably worse. Coincidence aside, it is known that about 10–20 percent of Parkinson's disease patients will develop dementia. If the dementing illness is apparent at the outset, management is more difficult. If such patients are given levodopa drugs for their parkinsonism symptoms, they can tolerate only small doses and are prone to side effects, particularly confused states and hallucinations. In other words, dementia limits the amount of levodopa it is possible to give, and control of parkinsonism symptoms is therefore less satisfactory.

The combination of Parkinson's disease and dementia is ultimately disabling. Families will need all the medical and social services possible to cope with the patient at home. Ultimately, periods in long-term hospitals or nursing homes may be necessary. However, research is being pursued actively in this area, and there is every hope that progress will be made.

KEY POINTS

- People with Parkinson's disease often feel anxious, apprehensive, or even depressed about their illness.
- Medical attention is needed early in depression.
- Confusion and hallucinations may be caused by sensitivity to antiparkinsonism drugs or by other unrelated illnesses.
- The combination of Parkinson's disease and dementia makes treatment difficult.

Disability in Parkinson's disease

If you have just been told that you have Parkinson's disease, you may feel gloomy and despondent. You may have visions of a shuffling, bent old person, see yourself in a wheelchair, and feel disheartened by the possibility of your family and friends having to look after your every need. These feelings are common, but in many cases they are unjustified by subsequent events.

BEING POSITIVE

It is important to understand the illness and put it into perspective. While it is true that some patients end up with severe physical and mental disabilities, many do not. A lot depends on how old you are when the condition is first diagnosed.

For example, if you have been fit and reasonably active and develop shaking in one hand in your 70s, it is safe to say that your life expectancy will not be reduced. Parkinsonism symptoms are unlikely to cause much disability before you are in your 80s. Even then, the

PRACTICAL HELP
Various aids, such as this wheeled walker, are available to help those who suffer from Parkinson's disease.

Hoehn and Yahr Scale for Rating Severity of Disability

The Hoehn and Yahr scale recognizes five distinct stages of Parkinson's disease.

STAGE 1
Unilateral disease only.

STAGE 2
Bilateral mild disease.

STAGE 3
Bilateral disease with early impairment of postural stability.

STAGE 4
Severe disease requiring considerable assistance.

STAGE 5
Confinement to bed or wheelchair unless aided.

symptoms may not be serious. Other coincidental illnesses, for example arthritis, bronchitis, heart disease, and stroke, are more likely to cause difficulties than Parkinson's disease.

If you are one of those people who has been afflicted when unusually young – in your 30s or 40s – the rate of deterioration is often slow. Although significant physical problems may eventually occur, you may well have many years of normal functioning and be able to continue both your professional work and your home life. Furthermore, new modifications of treatments are being developed rapidly, and, as a result, many more drugs are available now than 10 or 20 years ago. In addition, surgical techniques (see pp.59–61) are being used in certain cases, such as when drug treatment is no longer effective or the disease is advanced. The outlook is likely to continue to improve during the next decade.

DETERIORATION

In general, the course of the illness is a slow one. Sudden deterioration is unlikely unless brought about by another illness or by use of the wrong drugs. The disease remains stationary for 5–10 years or even longer in 15–20 percent of patients. Disabilities are mild and do not increase during this period. Why this is, we do not know.

MONITORING TREATMENT

The effects of treatment are vitally important in determining how much trouble the illness causes. The results of treatment are usually the most gratifying for the first several years. In order to assess the effectiveness of treatment or to determine the stage of the disease at any point in time, major problems, signs, and disabilities are noted. However, there are several different scales that are used for classifying the stages of the illness. The overall severity of the disease is rated using the established, although probably oversimplified, Hoehn and Yahr scale (see opposite page).

There are also detailed scales describing problems with walking, feeding, dressing, and other activities of daily living (ADL). The Unified Parkinson's Disease Rating Scale (UPDRS), the Northwestern University Disability Scale, and the King's College Hospital Scale are also commonly used.

The Webster score (see p.42) is a simpler scale for assessment and takes only 5–10 minutes to complete. It is used by doctors to record slowness of movement (bradykinesia), rigidity, tremor, gait, speech, and other signs of disease. It is composed of 10 items graded 0–3 each, producing scores of 0 (no signs of disability) to a maximum of 30 (most severe). There are two additional useful checks on the patient's balance and the ability to get up from a chair.

There are also scales for assessing dyskinesia (jerky, twitching movements). An example of such a scale is shown on page 43. By repeated use of these scales,

LOSING BALANCE
Poor balance is one of the symptoms assessed on scoring systems. Others include speech, tremor, posture, and slowness of movement.

Webster Score for the Assessment of Parkinson's Disease

The Webster scale is used by practitioners to assess the Parkinson's disease patient's overall pattern of symptoms. It takes about 5–10 minutes to complete the assessment.

STANDARD SYMPTOMS ASSESSED

Each item is graded according to a specific schedule, which is scored 0 (low) to 3 (high):

1	Bradykinesia of hands	6	Tremor
2	Rigidity	7	Facial expression
3	Posture	8	Seborrhea
4	Arm swing	9	Speech
5	Gait	10	Self-care

ADDITIONAL ITEMS SUGGESTED	**MENTAL STATE**
(scored 0 to 3)	(scored 0 to 3)
• Balance	• Confusion
• Rising from chair	• Hallucinosis
• Dyskinesia	• Dementia

the degree of improvement resulting from any form of treatment can be measured.

Just as the quality of life has been enhanced by drug treatment, so has the duration of life. Before the levodopa drugs were developed, the life expectancy after diagnosis was approximately 12 years. Many Parkinson's disease patients now have a normal life expectancy, and death is much more likely to be caused by unrelated common illnesses that affect the elderly.

Dyskinesia Scales

These specially designed scales are used by doctors in assessing the severity and duration of a Parkinson's disease patient's dyskinesia, or jerky, twitching movements.

A Duration: The percentage of time dyskinesia is present during waking hours:

0 = none
1 = 1–25 percent
2 = 26–50 percent
3 = 51–75 percent
4 = 76–100 percent

B Severity of dyskinesia

0 = noticeable, mild but not disabling
1 = mildly disabling
2 = moderately disabling
3 = severely disabling

NB: Additional scales from 0 to 3 can be used in the assessment of painful dyskinesia and dystonia.

KEY POINTS

- Not all Parkinson's disease patients end up with severe physical and mental disabilities.
- Specially designed scales are used to assess the severity of disability and the impact of treatment.
- Many patients now have a normal life expectancy.

Medical treatment

Treatment is aimed at abolishing the symptoms and disabilities caused by the illness as much as possible. We do not yet have drugs that will cure the disease or affect its natural progression. However, available drugs reverse the symptoms by replacing the essential chemicals, such as dopamine, necessary for normal transmission of nerve impulses and control of movements.

PART OF THE TREATMENT
Taking drugs is only part of the medical treatment for Parkinson's disease. Although the drugs used cannot prevent brain cell degeneration, they minimize the symptoms of the disorder.

━━ POINTS TO CONSIDER ━━

• Medical treatment should be customized to suit the needs of each individual patient and will need fine-tuning at intervals over the entire course of the illness. In Parkinson's disease, it is not enough to put the patient on a single pill, three times a day, and just leave it at that.

• Treatment should always be determined by symptoms and degree of disability. For example, at the onset, when the symptoms may be mild and inconspicuous, it is often best to give no drugs at all.

• Correct management of Parkinson's disease involves more than drugs alone. Active and positive efforts are necessary from you as well as from your partner or relatives. Assistance from primary care physicians, physical therapists, occupational therapists, and various other caregivers is also required at certain times in the disease.

SPECIALIST CARE

Most patients should be referred to a specialist, usually a neurologist, at an early stage of the disease in order to confirm the diagnosis and obtain advice about the immediate and future prospects of treatment. Patients are seen at intervals to assess their progress and drug treatment. Thereafter, the neurologist will arrange for regular follow-up at intervals that vary from two months to a year.

Chemical Imbalance in Parkinson's Disease

The levels of acetylcholine and dopamine in the brain are normally balanced. In Parkinson's disease, the cells that produce dopamine degenerate, resulting in an insufficient level of dopamine and relative overactivity of acetylcholine.

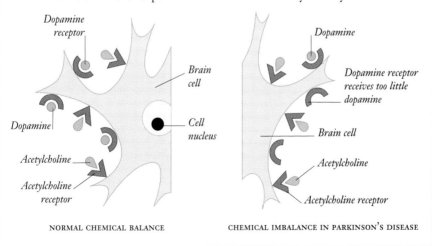

Dopamine receptor
Dopamine
Brain cell
Dopamine
Cell nucleus
Acetylcholine
Acetylcholine receptor

Dopamine receptor receives too little dopamine
Brain cell
Acetylcholine
Acetylcholine receptor

NORMAL CHEMICAL BALANCE

CHEMICAL IMBALANCE IN PARKINSON'S DISEASE

DRUG TREATMENT

Many neurologists start drug treatment with small doses of levodopa or a dopamine agonist. Anticholinergic drugs can be tried early if tremor is a predominant symptom.

Levodopa and dopamine agonists are the mainstay of drug treatment and are more effective than other drugs that are currently available. Several drugs are available as syrups and elixirs for patients who have difficulty swallowing pills or capsules. The striking benefits afforded by these drugs may, in some cases, slowly wear off after 5–10 years but still offer some relief. Patients' needs and responses to therapy vary widely.

One of the dopamine agonists may be used to supplement the levodopa treatment if it is not adequate.

Effect of Drugs Used in Parkinson's Disease

The balance between dopamine and acetylcholine in the brain can be restored by either a drug that blocks the acetylcholine receptors in the brain (an anticholinergic drug) or a dopamine-boosting drug, which increases dopamine activity.

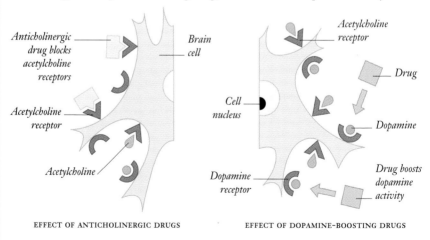

EFFECT OF ANTICHOLINERGIC DRUGS

EFFECT OF DOPAMINE-BOOSTING DRUGS

These drugs stimulate the dopamine receptors rather than supply more dopamine. Neurologists are now using dopamine agonists (bromocriptine, pergolide, pramipexole, and ropinirole) early in the course of treatment because they cause fewer jerky, twitching movements (dyskinesia) than levodopa, the drug most often used for established disease. However, most patients still require treatment with a levodopa drug within the first 3–4 years. Levodopa is converted in the brain to active dopamine.

Other drugs used in the treatment of Parkinson's disease include selegiline, tolcapone, and entacapone. Although selegiline is itself a weak antiparkinsonism drug, it is valuable during the early stages of the disease to control symptoms and delay by about one year the need for levodopa. Selegiline also reduces the wearing-off effects of levodopa that occur in the later stages of the disease (end-of-dose akinesia).

LEVODOPA DRUGS

These are the treatment of choice for moderate and severe Parkinson's disease. Rigidity, slowness, posture, and often tremor are improved by levodopa drugs. Their beneficial effects may be less marked in the elderly and in those with long-standing illness because such patients may be unable to tolerate a dose large enough to control their symptoms.

DRUG DOSE

Treatment is started with a low dose taken with food. This is gradually increased until the lowest dose necessary to produce acceptable control of symptoms and disability is reached.

Levodopa Drugs

Levodopa drugs are successful in treating most of the symptoms of moderate-to-severe Parkinson's disease. Dose requirements may vary greatly from patient to patient.

DRUG	TRADE NAME	SINGLE DOSE OF EACH COMPONENT
Levodopa with Carbidopa	Sinemet Sinemet CR	10/100 mg 25/100 mg

The pure form of levodopa has now been replaced by combinations of levodopa with carbidopa, which concentrates the levodopa in the brain and minimizes the side effects elsewhere in the body.

The best dose is often a compromise between near-total control of all symptoms and side effects. This usually requires the combination of low doses of several antiparkinsonism medications rather than high doses of a single drug. Many physicians like to keep a little in reserve in this way in case it is needed in the future. Most patients are untroubled by early side effects, although occasionally nausea, vomiting, or fainting may occur. These symptoms are often easily overcome by adjustments in dose and frequency.

SIDE EFFECTS

After several years on levodopa drugs, some patients develop abnormal jerky, twitching (choreic), or writhing (athetoid) movements called drug-induced dyskinesias. The side effects usually occur one to three hours after a dose when brain levels of dopamine are at their peak.

They affect the mouth, tongue, lips, and cheeks, and often the neck, the limbs, and the trunk. These side effects usually bother patients' spouses more often than they do the patients themselves because they are embarrassing rather than disabling. If severe, they can be reduced or even abolished by taking smaller doses of the drugs, which may then need to be administered more frequently. The usual response of Parkinson's disease and other kinds of symptomatic parkinsonism to levodopa and anticholinergic drugs is shown in the table on page 57.

The other most prominent unwanted side effects include mental disturbances such as confusion, disorientation, failing memory, and loss of concentration. As you grow older, abnormal movements or mental disturbances may make it necessary to reduce the dosage of levodopa. Although this may make you much calmer and more contented, it is likely to increase your parkinsonism symptoms – slowness and rigidity, difficulty walking, bent posture, and falls. In the end, most families find it easier to care for a patient who is slow, perhaps even immobile, but rational than for one who is more active but disoriented and confused.

Side Effects of Levodopa Drugs

Side effects are divided into those that occur initially and those that appear after a few years.

EARLY SIDE EFFECTS
(first few days and weeks):
Nausea and vomiting
Fainting

LATE SIDE EFFECTS (after 1–3 years)
Wearing-off at end of dose interval
Dyskinesia and dystonia
"On-off" fluctuations
Mental confusion and hallucinations

WEARING-OFF EFFECTS

At a later stage of Parkinson's disease, the duration of drug action seems shorter. You may notice wearing off at the end of each dose interval before the next dose is due (end-of-dose akinesia), or you may be aware of wearing off when you wake up each morning (early morning akinesia). Slowness, stiffness, and freezing are the most troublesome features. Sometimes a single dose does not work, often a dose that has been taken after lunch. In some cases, this is caused by proteins in the stomach and intestine from the preceding meal interfering with the absorption of the drug into the bloodstream. Modifying the diet may improve this problem.

The recently developed slow-release (controlled-release, or CR) preparations are effective for some patients. A single dose taken in the evening may reduce fitful sleep or the need to get up to use the bathroom during the night. The slow-release form of the medication may also control dystonic cramps in the legs and feet and may give you greater mobility when you first wake up in the morning, before the first dose of ordinary levodopa is taken. When it is used in this manner, the single dose of a controlled-release levodopa preparation at night should be used in combination with the usual daytime regimen of ordinary levodopa.

Slow-release Drugs
Controlled-release preparations can help to get rid of painful dystonic cramps in some patients.

An alternative regimen is to take the controlled-release preparation regularly in the daytime in place of shorter-acting levodopa. Levels of drug in the blood and brain tend to be lower and are achieved more slowly during the day. Therefore, the dose needs to be increased by about one-third above the previous levodopa dosage. This produces a smoother response of symptoms and shorter periods of immobility in the "off" phase. However, many patients find that they are never fully active or "on" and prefer the usual shorter-acting levodopa.

"On–off" Episodes

Later, "on–off" episodes may develop. The "on" phase occurs at peak dose, and the patient is then mobile and independent but often has abnormal dyskinetic movements. The "off" phase consists of sudden freezing, feet sticking to the floor, and immobility, sometimes accompanied by a feeling of fear and panic. Patients may suddenly switch from "on" to "off" and from "off" to "on"; the feeling has been compared to switching a light switch. This sensation is disconcerting and is sometimes mistakenly attributed to "nerves" or psychological problems. Lower, more frequent doses may ease this difficulty.

A related problem is painful cramplike twisting of the ankle and toes that often occurs at the end of a dose interval, just before the next dose is due, or sometimes at night. This is called drug-induced dystonia.

All these drug manipulations demand the patience and skill of both patient and physician. It is sometimes necessary to admit such patients to the hospital for specialized care and for frequent checks and ratings of symptoms, side effects, and dosage in order to achieve the fine-tuning for optimal performance. This process may take as long as one or two weeks.

DOPAMINE AGONISTS

It is common to introduce these drugs at an early stage, sometimes before levodopa, because they cause less dyskinesia than levodopa, and it is thought that they may delay the appearance of levodopa dyskinesias and fluctuations. Dopamine agonists may also be started when dyskinesias or "on–off" fluctuations develop.

Bromocriptine, pergolide, pramipexole, and ropinirole are all dopamine agonists. If one agonist fails or is not tolerated, another can be tried. When used with levodopa, they reduce the wearing-off time and may allow a reduction in levodopa dose.

These drugs are started in small doses and slowly increased every week or so until benefit is apparent without undue side effects. It may take 2–3 months to find the best stable dose. When the dopamine agonist is taken in combination with levodopa, it may be possible to reduce the levodopa dose by about 25

Dopamine Agonists

This chart lists the commonly used dopamine agonists, together with their trade names and typical dosages. Their effect is to stimulate activity of the dopamine receptors.

DRUG	TRADE NAME	SINGLE DOSE	DOSE PER DAY
Bromocriptine	Parlodel	1, 2.5, 5, or 10 mg	20–30 mg
Pergolide	Permax	50, 250, or 1,000 mcg	750–4,000 mcg
Ropinirole	Requip	0.25, 1, 2, or 5 mg	12–20 mg
Pramipexole	Mirapex	0.125, 0.25, 0.5, 1, or 1.5 mg	2–4 mg

*Note: 1,000 micrograms (mcg) = 1 milligram (mg)

percent when the benefit becomes apparent. In general, patients with severe vascular, kidney, or liver disease, or those who are pregnant or breast-feeding, should not take this group of drugs.

SIDE EFFECTS

Dopamine agonists are strong drugs that reduce all the symptoms of Parkinson's disease, but their side effects can be serious. They cause more severe psychiatric complications of confusion, delusions, and frank aggressive behavior in a number of patients. These are usually reversible by reducing the dose, but it is often necessary to stop the drug. These psychiatric complications are especially likely in those over 70 and in those with previous confusion or dementia. Dopamine agonists can also aggravate stomach ulcers and arterial disease in the legs. In general, they should not be given to older patients and should always be supervised by a specialist.

ANTICHOLINERGIC DRUGS

These drugs are valuable for treating early tremor and rigidity but are not as effective as levodopa in treating slowness, freezing, and falls. They are good at controlling salivation and drooling because they cause dry mouth. They work well with levodopa drugs but are usually tapered gradually in older patients or if there is a tendency to confusion, hallucinations, or memory impairment. Symptoms from an enlarged prostate gland or liability to glaucoma may be worsened. Anticholinergics are especially helpful in drug-induced parkinsonism states and rare postencephalitic cases. Recommended doses have similar potencies and side effects.

Anticholinergic Drugs

These drugs may be used to treat Parkinson's disease in its early stage, when the symptoms are mild and tremor predominates. They are generally used in younger patients who do not have the added complications of the elderly.

DRUG	TRADE NAME	SINGLE DOSE	DOSE RANGE PER DAY
Orphenadrine	Norflex	100 mg	200 mg
	Norflex (injection)	60 mg/2 ml	60–120 mg
	Norgesic	25 mg	75–200 mg
	Norgesic Forte	50 mg	75–200 mg
Trihexyphenidyl	Artane	2 or 5 mg	6–15 mg
	Artane (elixir)	2 mg/5 ml	
Benztropine	Cogentin	0.5, 1, or 2 mg	0.5–6 mg
	Cogentin (injection)	1 mg/1 ml	

OTHER DRUGS

In addition to the drug groups already described, several other medications may be used instead of or in combination with levodopa at various stages in the disease.

SELEGILINE

Selegiline is a weak antiparkinsonism drug, but it slightly strengthens the effects of levodopa drugs and may reduce "on–off" swings, especially the immobility that is experienced during the "off" phase. It is best given early in the illness, since it may temporarily delay the need for other drugs, such as levodopa.

The early reports that selegiline had a protective effect by slowing down the disease remain controversial. A dose of 5 mg twice daily is well tolerated, and side effects are uncommon. One group of British researchers found a slightly increased mortality rate and a tendency to fainting attacks (syncope) in some patients treated with selegiline, although most published studies do not show such effects. No reason for this possible finding has been discovered, and, since a causal link is not yet established, most physicians continue to prescribe the drug in standard dosages.

Other Drugs

Typical doses of four other drugs commonly used to treat Parkinson's disease are shown in this chart.

DRUG	TRADE NAME	DOSE	DOSE PER DAY
Amantadine	Symmetrel Symmetrel (syrup)	100 mg 50 mg/5 ml	200 mg
Selegiline	Eldepryl	10 mg	5–10 mg
Tolcapone	Tasmar	100 mg/ 200 mg	300 mg/ 600 mg
Entacapone		200 mg with each dose of levodopa	

TOLCAPONE AND ENTACAPONE

Of the many new drugs being assessed, tolcapone and entacopone work by inhibiting an enzyme (catechol-O-methyltransferase, or COMT) that breaks down levodopa, thus prolonging its duration of action. This group of drugs improves motor function (strength and co-ordinated movements), lengthens the duration of the "on" phase, and reduces the necessary levodopa dosage. Since tolcapone has been associated with liver enzyme elevations, a blood test is required every two weeks.

AMANTADINE

Amantadine is weakly anticholinergic and has few side effects. This substance has mild dopamine-releasing properties that boost dopamine levels. It is generally used in patients with mild Parkinson's disease to alleviate tremor and, to a lesser extent, rigidity and bradykinesia. It is also occasionally used in patients with more advanced disease. Recent studies have suggested that it may help suppress involuntary movement in patients with levodopa-related complications.

DRUG WARNINGS

Certain drugs should not be used in Parkinson's disease, such as phenothiazine tranquilizers, antipsychotic drugs, and certain drugs for stomach ailments (metoclopramide, prochlorperazine). You should never take monoamine oxidase (type A) inhibitors for depression, but tricyclic antidepressants and selective serotonin reuptake inhibitors (SSRIs) can be used when needed.

How Parkinson's Disease Responds to Drugs

This table shows the usual response of Parkinson's disease and other kinds of symptomatic parkinsonism to levodopa and anticholinergic drugs.

CONDITION	LEVODOPA	ANTICHOLINERGIC DRUGS
Parkinson's disease	● ● ●	● ●
Drug-induced parkinsonism	● ●	● ●
Multiple-system atrophies, including progressive supranuclear palsy	+/-	+/-
Other causes of parkinsonism	+/-	+/-

KEY	● ● ● usually very good	● ● moderate	+/- variable response

57

KEY POINTS

- Drug treatment reverses the symptoms of Parkinson's disease by replacing the essential chemicals necessary for normal transmission of nerve impulses and control of movements.
- Drugs are chosen to match the stage of the disease and need adjustments at intervals throughout the illness.
- Combinations of levodopa and carbidopa are the most effective.
- Unwanted side effects can be reduced or abolished by altering the drug dose and frequency of administration.
- When wearing-off effects of drugs are troublesome, the recently developed slow-release (controlled-release, or CR) preparations are useful in some patients.
- Dopamine agonists should be given with caution to older patients and should always be supervised by a specialist.

Surgery for Parkinson's disease

Surgery may be used in place of drug treatment to treat motor complications that result either from long-standing drug therapy or advanced disease.

SURGERY

Surgery has recently experienced a resurgence of importance in the treatment of Parkinson's disease. Despite the availability of a variety of medications for treating Parkinson's disease and the on-going development of new drugs, many patients eventually develop motor complications that result from either long-standing drug therapy or advanced disease. New surgical techniques have enabled physicians to locate precise targets in the brain and either create lesions or place stimulators in those regions that may contribute to the symptoms of parkinsonism.

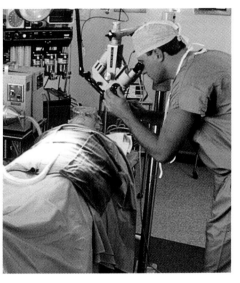

SURGICAL TREATMENT
Research into new surgical treatments for Parkinson's disease is continuing.

NEUROABLATION

The goal of neuroablation is to disrupt an abnormally functioning structure in a way that leaves normal voluntary movement intact. Using both MRI technology and microelectrode recording, neurosurgeons can locate the precise position of deep brain structures and then destroy nerve cells that are functioning abnormally. A procedure called ventrolateral thalamotomy has been very effective in suppressing tremor that is not responsive to medication. More recently, physicians have been placing lesions in a part of the brain called the globus pallidus interna for relief of the symptoms of Parkinson's disease and the involuntary movements caused by medications used to treat the disease. This procedure, called a pallidotomy, can also reduce tremor and rigidity. Both thalamotomy and pallidotomy have some risk of neurologic complications and should be discussed thoroughly with your doctor before they are considered.

DEEP-BRAIN STIMULATION

In deep-brain stimulation, an electrode is placed into a target site in the brain through a small opening in the skull, known as a burr hole. This electrode is then attached to a pacemaker-like generator, which is usually placed under the skin near the collarbone. The electrode, in a fashion similar to that of a cardiac pacemaker, can block the abnormal neuron activity and function similarly to a neuroablative procedure. Deep-brain stimulation has the advantage of being "reversible" because no permanent lesion is made in the brain. The technique alters the function of an abnormal part of the brain rather than destroying tissue. Performed on the thalamus, this method has been very effective at alleviating tremor. More recently, deep-brain stimulation of other brain regions, such as the globus pallidus and subthalamic nucleus, has been effective in reducing tremor, muscle rigidity, and uneven gait in some patients.

THE FUTURE

The use of neuroablation and deep-brain stimulation is likely to expand with recent studies designed to determine the precise effects of these procedures. In the long term, therapies aimed at altering the course of Parkinson's disease itself will become the standard of care. While the use of fetal cells and other tissue transplants has been controversial and the results inconclusive, there is a flurry of research into other sources of tissue transplantation and gene therapy approaches that will likely prove effective at altering the progression of this common affliction.

KEY POINTS

- Surgery may be used if drug treatment is not effective. The procedures most commonly used place lesions or stimulators in the affected area of the brain.
- Neuroablation involves the destruction of nerve cells that are functioning abnormally.
- Deep-brain stimulation blocks abnormal nerve activity by the action of an implanted electrode.

General management

Drug treatment is the most important single measure in reversing the symptoms and disabilities of Parkinson's disease, but there is far more to the treatment of the patient than just the administration of drugs.

Many problems that are faced by patients are not caused by Parkinson's disease but by the coincidental conditions from which many people suffer and which may

SPECIALIST CARE
Your primary care physician will be interested in your total care because you may have other conditions that require medical treatment.

require medical attention. Patients may have diabetes, high blood pressure, asthma, heart disease, bronchitis, or arthritis. It is essential, therefore, that the doctor, whether your primary care physician or a specialist, does not ignore other medical conditions and treat only the symptoms of Parkinson's disease.

IDENTIFYING THE PROBLEMS

Certain problems occur commonly in Parkinson's disease, and the first step is to identify them before outlining plans to correct them. Common problems in

movement that you may have noticed include:
- Walking slowly.
- Walking with short, shuffling steps.
- Walking through doorways causes you to stop or hesitate.
- Your feet seem to freeze to the floor.
- Handwriting smaller, shaky, and spidery.
  You may encounter difficulty in:
- Turning in a narrow space without falling.
- Swinging the arms automatically when walking.
- Getting out of a chair.
- Standing straight instead of hunched forward.
- Turning over in bed.
- Getting on and off the toilet.
- Fine hand manipulations, such as those involved in dressing and undressing.
- Using a screwdriver or sewing on buttons.

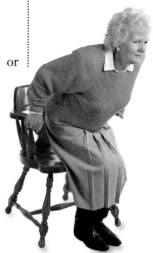

MOBILITY PROBLEMS
Simple physical movements such as getting out of a chair may become increasingly difficult for the Parkinson's disease sufferer.

PHYSICAL THERAPY

Physical therapy has specific benefits for specific problems. It also has a generally beneficial effect on morale by assuring the patient that something positive is being done and that he or she is playing an active part in the treatment. The motivation, personality, and attitude of both patient and therapist have a marked influence on the success of therapy. Bad habits are eradicated more easily if they are caught early. Later on, motivation may be poor, memory and concentration impaired, and effective cooperation may be impossible.

Assessment of the condition is the first step. This includes determination of:
- Physical disabilities.
- Learning capacity and mental state.

• Home circumstances.

• The availability of friends and family members to continue to help.

EXERCISES

Exercises and activity are important because they mobilize joints and muscles, lessen stiffness, and improve posture. They aim to:

• Correct abnormal gait.

• Correct bad posture.

• Prevent or minimize stiffness and contractures of the muscles and tendons.

• Improve use and facilities of the limbs.

• Provide a regimen that can be used at home by the patient.

Regular exercise is beneficial whenever disabilities permit. It helps maintain muscle tone and strength and prevent contractures and stiffening. Walking is one of the most valuable exercises. Most people in the early stages of Parkinson's disease can walk a mile or two each day, sometimes much more. A conscious effort should be made to keep the back straight, the shoulders back, and the head upright, and to take long, slow strides. Even more severely affected people can often walk 300 or 400 yards and perhaps repeat this once or twice every day. Slippery surfaces, snow, ice, and wet leaves obviously should be avoided.

The physical therapist will concentrate on teaching you to sit straight, often in a high upright chair, aided by a cushion behind your back. He or she will show you how to focus on striking your heels down when walking, and how to rise from a sitting position to a standing one more easily by pulling your heels in under the front edge of the chair and throwing your weight forward as you get up. Standing in front of a long mirror may help you see and correct any stooped or bent posture of your neck and trunk.

SELF-MOTIVATION

Exercises must be repeated constantly and practiced at home, particularly when the therapist is not present. The exercise sessions may be made easier and more rhythmic and pleasant if they are accompanied by music. Participation in outpatient therapy may be helpful, and encouragement may be derived from group exercise sessions. Therapeutic vacations that include vigorous activity can also be arranged through one of the associations that deal specifically with this disease (see Useful addresses, p.73).

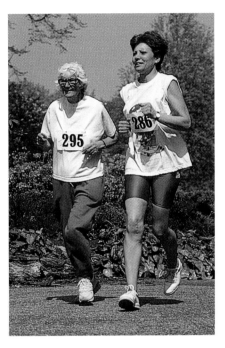

VIGOROUS EXERCISE
With regular practice, some patients find themselves able to undertake quite strenuous exercise, and specially tailored therapeutic vacations are possible.

OCCUPATIONAL THERAPY

A wide range of home aids are available, many through your HMO or insurance plan, although you may need to purchase some of them yourself. A home visit by an occupational therapist is invaluable, and he or she will identify specific problems and determine the need for specific apparatus, such as handrails and high seats. Wide handles on faucets, antislip kitchen surfaces, lever arms on taps, raised working surfaces in the kitchen and greenhouse, and Velcro fasteners on garments and shoes are examples of the means by which you can make your activities easier and regain your independence.

APPLIANCES

As the disease progresses, some patients require aids to activity. Canes enhance your stability and are socially unobtrusive. A four-point cane provides a wider base. Walkers are not recommended, except as a short-term measure when you are mobilizing after injury or operation in the hospital, because they break the natural rhythm of walking. However, if they are fitted with wheels, they can be helpful. Delta frames, which have two "legs" and a front wheel, or a rotator with two legs and two wheels are helpful. Brakes add to your sense of security.

Individual exercises are intended to help your balance, increase your stride, and perhaps relieve the pain of a frozen shoulder, which is a common complication.

Manual dexterity may be improved by practice with blocks, jigsaw puzzles, and certain games. Grab rails fitted near your bed and in the bathroom are helpful. Buttons and zippers can be replaced by Velcro fasteners. Casual or elastic-sided shoes or sneakers may be much better than shoes with laces.

Large-handled knives, forks, and spoons, and stick-on plates can prevent spills. Many can be supplied or recommended by the physical or occupational therapist.

A good liaison between the hospital-based physical therapist and occupational therapist, the social worker, and your health-care providers is an enormous advantage. They will discuss assessments and plans when you are admitted to the hospital, and will continue supervision after you go home.

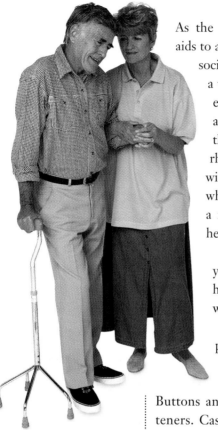

INCREASING MOBILITY
Walking aids, such as the one shown here, can help to promote independence in the Parkinson's disease patient.

SPEECH THERAPY

Many patients are embarrassed and frustrated by their speech. You may find that you speak quietly, are unable to shout, and that friends are always asking you to repeat yourself or speak up. Speech may be slurred and hesitant with lack of variation in pitch and volume.

Speech therapists can assess the way you breathe and move your lips, tongue, and jaw in the formation of speech – all actions that we normally perform unconsciously.

In Parkinson's disease, the voice box (larynx) no longer works properly, producing a monotonous pitch, lack of volume control, and lack of stress on certain sounds. Your voice may sound hoarse, quiet, and monotonous. Speech therapy may use audio feedback in which you hear your own speech after a measured interval. This can modify and improve your voice and speech output. This and other measures can, to a modest extent, help retrain the voice and speech, but dramatic improvements are not common. In some instances, collagen injections into the vocal cords may augment speech volume.

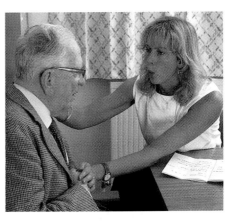

IMPROVING SPEECH
Speech therapy can give some help in retraining the voice and speech of a patient, but improvements may be limited.

COMMUNICATION AIDS

Aids to communication include Edu-Com Scanning, a device that points to a word or picture showing your intention and meaning. "Micro-writer" links a TV, printer, or speech synthesizer and can be of occasional help to patients when speech training is unsuccessful. A personal computer may help you write letters, perform

67

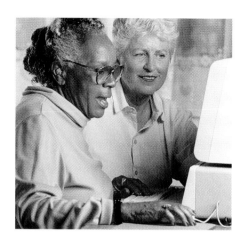

WRITING AID
For patients who find writing difficult, a small home computer may prove an invaluable aid.

business activities, and attend to your finances at home. Modern computer programs are fairly easy to learn, and there is a wide range of recreational games and educational material that may occupy your time and expand your interests.

DIET

Patients with Parkinson's disease do not require a special diet but should have a balanced, enjoyable diet with meat, fish, fruit, and vegetables, like anyone else. Sometimes, a dose of levodopa does not work, particularly after lunch. This may occur because proteins in the stomach and intestine from the preceding meal can interfere with the absorption of the drug into the bloodstream. Your specialist may advise you to have a low-protein lunch with small amounts of meat, fish, poultry, eggs, or cheese, but to include more of these foods in your main evening meal.

GENERAL OBSERVATIONS

With the help of your primary care physician, you should obtain up-to-date medical support and supervision of your drug and physical treatment and advice about any possible side effects. More specialized guidance is available from consulting neurologists, who should supervise the care of most patients with Parkinson's disease when possible. Welfare services and hospital units also provide the support of physical therapists, occupational therapists, and social workers when the need arises.

Activity throughout the illness is crucial. Do as much as you can, but be sensible and do not overexert to the point of exhaustion. Three walks of 400 yards each are nearly as beneficial as one of 1,200 yards. You will also have to make certain adjustments in your lifestyle, but these are usually obvious, and changes are gradual to allow you plenty of time to make these alterations. You may have to allow a little more time to get dressed or get to work or to plan and pack for vacations or trips. It may take two tries instead of one to mow the lawn. Try not to let this irritate you. A little planning ahead and allowing more time will make most tasks possible.

Do not get fanatical about miraculous cures that you read about or gossip that you hear. A lot of money can be spent on false remedies, health foods, and other unorthodox therapies. Medical opinion has no rooted objection to some complementary therapies, but physicians do not generally use them unless they have been carefully and scientifically tested so that it is clear that they are beneficial.

CONCLUSIONS

Although there has been considerable progress in the last few years, Parkinson's disease remains something of an enigma. We know that there is degeneration of certain small but vital areas of the brain, and that it is not a condition caused by aging. Its causes are complex, but the major one is a lack of the essential chemical transmitter, dopamine, which can be effectively replaced by modern drug treatment. This permits a full and active life for many years after onset of the disease.

Medical and social research is funded on a large scale by Parkinson's disease foundations and by other organizations. As a result, hardly a year goes by without some important additional knowledge – additions that are of practical importance to each and every sufferer of Parkinson's disease.

All new discoveries require careful scientific scrutiny before they can be accepted as valid. There are many avenues of progress under investigation.

Although we are dealing with a slowly progressing illness in most cases, you should remember that most patients have a normal life span that allows many years of activity and enjoyment. Sufferers of Parkinson's disease can face the future with measured optimism.

KEY POINTS

- An exercise program can be developed with the help of a physical therapist.
- Many aids are available to encourage independence in the home.
- Speech may be improved by working with a speech therapist.
- Patients should eat a healthy, balanced diet, but no special diet is necessary.

Questions and answers

What causes Parkinson's disease?

We do not know the cause. Investigations have sought environmental factors such as contaminants of food, water, and air and exposure to poisonous chemicals at work but have failed to produce an answer. Although there is a weak hereditary factor, it is not the cause but may make certain people more susceptible to unidentified substances to which we may be exposed.

I have been under a lot of stress. Could that be the cause?

No. Stress and tension may cause a temporary worsening of symptoms, but they do not cause the disease. Depression is a common problem in Parkinson's disease and may reduce your general efficiency, drive, and ability to cope. However, it is generally much improved by antidepressant drugs.

Will I pass it on to my children or grandchildren?

Although there is a slightly higher incidence of perhaps 1 in 20 cases in close relatives, Parkinson's disease is not an inherited disease.

I have heard that selegiline will slow down the disease. Should I take it?

It remains uncertain whether or not selegiline affects the disease process in the brain. It is, nonetheless, useful early in the illness and acts by relieving early symptoms, thereby delaying the time when it becomes necessary to start levodopa drugs. Side effects are infrequent and mild.

Is there any advantage in delaying the start of levodopa drugs?

It is generally thought sensible not to start levodopa before symptoms are more severe and are beginning to interfere with work and leisure, although there is no clinical evidence that the early use of levodopa is harmful. There is no advantage in delaying levodopa once symptoms begin to interfere with social or occupational function.

What will be the effects of levodopa, and will it have side effects?

After starting levodopa, stiffness, slowness of movements, walking difficulties, and posture usually improve. Shaking does not always disappear but may be reduced. Benefits continue to increase as the fine-tuning of dose and timing is carefully monitored. A few patients have nausea or faintness in the first few weeks, but taking pills on a full stomach and starting with small doses and increasing slowly will usually improve this. Abnormal movements, fluctuations in effects before and after each dose, and mental problems can develop later in the illness, but adjustments of drugs and dosage often improve or abolish these symptoms.

I have taken dopamine for two years. Why am I now getting these funny twitching movements?

Your movements are probably dyskinesias or dystonias caused by a slight overspill or excess of drug on the sensitive receptors in the brain. They usually occur some 30–60 minutes after each dose and last for a few minutes. Your doctor may recommend a slight reduction in dose given at shorter intervals. A controlled-release (CR) preparation or the addition of a dopamine agonist helps some patients.

Why is it taking so long for the pills to work, and why do they wear off so quickly?

After a few years the brain does not absorb or distribute levodopa as efficiently, and the dopamine receptors do not respond quite as effectively as at the start of treatment. Alteration by your physician of the dose and frequency and the addition of other medications often overcome this problem.

I find that I cannot concentrate or remember things as I used to. Is Parkinson's disease responsible?

Memory and concentration often diminish with normal aging, irrespective of Parkinson's disease. If you have become depressed, this can also affect concentration and memory but often improves with simplification of or additional drug therapy. Only a small percentage of Parkinson's disease sufferers become demented.

Am I likely to benefit from surgery?

Motor complications may develop due to either long-standing drug treatment or advanced disease. Patients thus affected may benefit from new surgical techniques that enable surgeons to locate precise targets in the brain and place either lesions or stimulators in the areas that may contribute to the symptoms of parkinsonism.

Useful addresses

Parkinson's Disease Foundation
Online: www.pdf.org
710 West 168th Street
New York, NY 10032
Tel: (800) 457-6676
Tel: (212) 923-4700

American Parkinson's Disease Association
Online: www.apdaparkinson.com
1250 Hylan Blvd. Suite 4B
Staten Island, NY 10305
Tel: (800) 223-2732
Tel: (718) 981-8001

National Parkinson Foundation
Online: www.parkinson.org
1501 NW 9th Avenue
Bob Hope Road
Miami, FL 33136
Tel: (800) 327-4545

The Parkinson's Institute
Online: www.parkinsoninstitute.org
1170 Morse Avenue
Sunnyvale, CA 94089-1605
Tel: (408) 734-2800
E-mail: outreach@parkinsoninstitute.org

Parkinson's Support Group of America
11376 Cherry Hill Road #204
Beltsville, MD 20705
Tel: (301) 937-1545

Parkinson's Action Network
Online: www.sonic.net
818 College Avenue, Suite C
Santa Rosa, CA 95404
Tel: (800) 850-4726
Tel: (707) 544-1994
E-mail: pan@sonic.net

Young Parkinson's Support Network of California
APDA Young Parkinson's I & R Center
1041 Foxenwood Drive
Santa Monica, CA 93455
Tel: (800) 223-9776
Tel: (805) 934-2216

National Institute of Neurological Disease and Stroke
Online: www.nids.nih.gov
PO Box 5801
Bethesda, MD 20824
Tel: (800) 352-9424
E-mail: nindswebadmin@nih.gov

Notes

Notes

Notes

Notes

Index

A

acetylcholine 13–14, 45, 46
  see also anticholinergic
    drugs
aging 8, 16
akinesia 23, 47, 49–50
Alzheimer's disease 31, 37
amantadine (Symmetrel) 55, 56
anticholinergic drugs 53–4, 57
  disease response 46, 53, 57
  dopamine–acetylcholine
    imbalance 14, 45
  side effects 35
antidepressants 34
appliances 66–8
apraxia 36
assessment scales 40, 41–3

B

balance 24, 42
basal ganglia 11–15
benign essential tremor 29
bladder habits 24–5, 40
bowel habits 24
bradykinesia 23, 41
brain 11–17, 19–21
bromocriptine 47, 52

C

carbidopa 8
  CR preparations 48
  dosage 48
  side effects 48
causes 8, 11–17, 71
cogwheel rigidity 22
computers 67–8
concentration 49, 63, 72
confusion 35–6, 42, 48, 52
constipation 25

consultants 10, 28–9
contraindications, drug
  therapy 56
controlled-release (CR)
  preparations 48, 50, 72

D

deep-brain stimulation 60–1
dementia 31, 37
depression 33–4
deterioration 40
diagnosis 9, 28–31
diet 50, 68
disabilities 39–43, 62–4
dopamine 9
  acetylcholine 13–14, 45–6
  agonists 46–7, 51–3, 72
  drug treatments 44–7
  MPTP poisoning 19–21
  receptors 15, 16
  substantia nigra 12–13
dopamine–acetylcholine
  imbalance 13, 14
dosages 72
  anticholinergic drugs 54
  dopamine agonists 52–3
  levodopa 47–8, 50
  selegiline 55
drooling 26
drug-induced parkinsonism
  18–19
drug treatments 44–58
  antidepressants 34
  contraindications 56
  dopamine agonists 46–7,
    51–3, 72
  see also anticholinergic
    drugs; levodopa drugs;
    side effects

dyskinesia 41–3, 47, 48–50,
  52, 72
dystonia 43, 49, 51, 72

E

Edu-Com Scanning 67
Eldepryl *see* selegiline
entacopone 47, 55, 56
exercise, physical 64–5

F

facial appearance 25, 42
festination 24
fluoxetine (Prozac) 34
forgetfulness 31, 35

G

gene therapy 61
general management 62–70
genetic etiology 16
glutathione 14

H

hallucinations 35–6, 49
hand symptoms 13, 22, 29, 39,
  63
handwriting 23, 29
heredity 16, 71
Hoehn and Yahr Scale 40–1

I

incontinence 24–5

L

levodopa drugs 9, 47–51
  delaying prescription 71
  dementia 37
  diet 72
  dosage 47–8, 50
  on–off episodes 49, 51

selegiline 47, 54–5
  side effects 35, 48–9, 72
  wearing-off effects 47,
    49–51
Lewy body disease 21, 31
life expectancy 8, 43

M

medical treatment 44–58
  depression 34
  effectivity 42–3
  gene therapy 61
  neurologist 10, 28–9, 45
  physical therapies 10, 63–5
  surgery 59–61
  see also drug treatments
memory lapses 31, 35, 72
Micro-Writer 67
micrographia 23
mitochondrial complex I 14,
  21
movement
  akinesia 23
  automatic 13, 25, 26
  bradykinesia 23
  dyskinesia 41–3, 4, 48–50,
    52, 72
MPTP 19–21
multiple sclerosis 30
multiple-system atrophies 21

N

nerve cells 11–16
neuroablation 59–60, 61
neuroleptics 18–19, 20
neurologist 10, 28–9, 45

O

occupational therapy 9, 65–6
on–off episodes 49, 51

P

pain 26
Parkinson, James 18
paroxitene 34
Paxil *see* paroxitene
pergolide 47
physical therapies 10, 63–5
poison-induced parkinsonism
  19–21
postencephalitic parkinsonism
  19
posture 22, 23–4, 40
pramipexole 47, 52
prevalence 8
primary care physician 10, 45
progressive supranuclear palsy
  21
Prozac *see* fluoxetine
psychological issues 32–8
  concentration 72
  confusion 35–6
  dementia 31, 37
  depression 33–4
  memory 31, 35, 72

R

rigidity 22, 23
ropinirole 47, 52

S

selegiline (Eldepryl) 47,
  54–5, 71
sertraline 34
side effects
  confusion 35, 36
  dopamine agonists 53
  levodopa drugs 35, 48–9, 72
  neuroleptics 18–19, 20
  selegiline 55
signs 7, 22–7

Sinemet *see* carbidopa
slow-release preparations 48,
  50, 72
speech difficulties 25–6
speech therapy 9, 67
stress 71
strokes 30–1
substantia nigra 11–13, 16,
  21
surgery 59–61
swallowing 25–6
Symmetrel *see* amantadine
symptomatic parkinsonism
  18–21
symptoms 7–8, 22–7, 40
  akinesia 23
  balance 24, 42
  drug treatments 47
  posture 22, 23–4, 40
  psychological 32–8, 72
  rigidity 22, 23
  tremor 22, 23, 29

T

tolcapone 47, 55, 56
tremor 22, 23, 29
twin studies 16
types of parkinsonism
  18–21

W

walking 23, 24, 64
wearing-off effects 49–51
Webster score 41, 42

Z

Zoloft *see* sertraline

Acknowledgments

PUBLISHER'S ACKNOWLEDGMENTS
Dorling Kindersley Publishing, Inc. would like to thank the following for their help
and participation in this project:

Managing Editor Stephanie Jackson; **Managing Art Editor** Nigel Duffield;
Editorial Assistance Judit Z. Bodnar, Janel Bragg, Alrica Goldstein, Mary Lindsay,
Irene Pavitt, Jennifer Quasha, Design Revolution;
Design Assistance Sarah Hall, Marianne Markham, Design Revolution, Chris Walker;
Production Michelle Thomas, Elizabeth Cherry.

Consultancy Dr. Tony Smith, Dr. Sue Davidson;
Indexing Indexing Specialists, Hove; **Administration** Christopher Gordon.

Organizations St. John's Ambulance, St. Andrew's Ambulance Organization,
British Red Cross.

Picture Research Angela Anderson, Andy Sansom;
Picture Librarian Charlotte Oster.

PICTURE CREDITS
The publisher would like to thank the following for their kind
permission to reproduce their photographs. Every effort has been made
to trace the copyright holders. Dorling Kindersley apologizes for any
unintentional omissions and would be pleased, in any such cases,
to add an acknowledgment in future editions.

Sally & Richard Greenhill Photo Library p.34, p.65;
Robert Harding p. 7, p.68 (Patrick Ramsey); **Science Photo Library** p.18 (Gary Watson),
p.26 (Tirot/BSIP), p.59 (Stevie Grand), p.67 (Hattie Young).